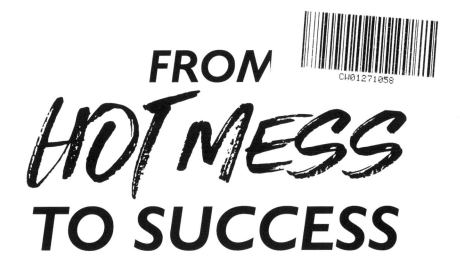

FROM HOT MESS TO SUCCESS

A Wild Woman's Guide to Claiming Your Freedom and Taking Back Control of Your Life!

GEORGINA NOEL

First published in 2020 by Georgina Noel

© Georgina Noel
The moral rights of the author have been asserted.
This book is a SpiritCast Network of Books

Author:
    Noel, Georgina

Title:
    From Hot Mess To Success; A Wild Woman's Guide to Claiming Your Freedom and Taking Back Control of Your Life!

ISBN:
    979-8-61917-764-0

All rights reserved. Except as permitted under the Australian Copyright Act 1968 (for example, a fair dealing for the purposes of study, research, criticism or review), no part of this book may be reproduced, stored in a retrieval system, communicated or transmitted in any form or by any means without prior written permission. All enquiries should be made to the publisher at gnoel1983@gmail.com

Editor-in-chief: Anita Saunders
Cover Design: Sarah Rose Graphic Design

Disclaimer:
The material in this publication is of the nature of general comment only, and does not represent professional advice. It is not intended to provide specific guidance for particular circumstances and it should not be relied on as the basis for any decision to take action or not take action on any matter which it covers. Readers should obtain professional advice where appropriate, before making any such decision. To the maximum extent permitted by law, the author and publisher disclaim all responsibility and liability to any person, arising directly or indirectly from any person taking or not taking action based on the information in this publication.

FROM HOT MESS TO SUCCESS

A Wild Woman's Guide to Claiming Your Freedom and Taking Back Control of Your Life!

So I'm walking through the woods. It's a Bank Holiday Monday and I'm walking through the woods looking like a crazy fuck, mascara stained down my cheeks, not even sure why I bother putting it on anymore, maybe just so people will stop fucking asking me if I'm okay and treating me like a piece of fucking glass: "Be careful with her, she's very delicate at the moment." [laughs a little too manically]

Delicate, fragile: FUCK YOU!

I'm running now.

"Which one is it? Where are you? I can't feel you. [breaks down] I can't feel you anymore."

Running to the nearest tree, I grab it and plead for its help.

"Help me find him. Please God, if you're up there, please help me find him."

I'm not sure what a fucking tree was going to do to help, but suddenly I was filled with a ferocious certainty.

Eyes wide. I turn.

"I'm coming, Fran, I'm coming for you."

I turn and run back the way I've come through the woods. Passersby walking their dogs, their children skipping, laughing, and swinging on that fucking swing.

I wonder if he ever swung on that swing.

All these people with their stupid fucking smiles and their stupid fucking lives. Don't they know? Have they not been made aware that the world has fucking ended and we're all just waiting for our turn now …

INTRODUCTION

What you have just read is an excerpt from a short play I wrote about an actual experience of me hunting through the woods in which my friend hanged himself, trying to find the tree where he did it. After he died, I was obsessed. I couldn't think about ANYTHING else. I used it as a reason to completely stall my life and, though now I understand why this needed to happen, back then I was a complete Hot Mess. I was like a woman possessed.

In case you're wondering, I did find the EXACT tree as I found out the next day from a police officer.

I am getting WAY ahead of myself here though, so let me ease you in. Well, I say EASE YOU IN, but that's not really my style. I've never been one for small talk!

I was inspired to write this book because I work with a lot of people, predominantly women, who struggle to step into their power and own their voice in the world and they stifle themselves for fear of what other people will think of them. I myself have had a huge journey with self-expression and releasing the giving of fucks about the opinions of others and it has been incredibly liberating.

My aim is to ignite in you the passion and fire to take charge of your life and fulfil your potential. One of my genuine biggest fears is that I would never reach my TRUE potential and when I see other women playing small or hiding from the world and themselves, I just wanna swoop in and show them how incredible they are and how much magic they have inside of them, that they are perfect and there is nothing fucking wrong with them.

The main message of this book is: YOU are the only person who can change your life and create what you want in the world so stop outsourcing your power and let's get you on track for cracking open the life of your dreams!

This book is for sassy-ass women who are fed up with reading fluffy spiritual bullshit and want a kick up the butt – women like us like our spirituality with a healthy side dose of gangster.

You're likely feeling frustrated and disempowered by life. You're seeking to take charge of it and ready to understand why the fuck bad shit keeps happening to you. You KNOW you have so much potential and feel underappreciated. Take this book as a sign; let it be the catalyst that sparks the fire in you! I want to remind you who you really are.
I know you take on a lot of responsibility and you want everyone to be happy, but you haven't fully owned that YOUR happiness is the most important thing.

During our time together, you will release the guilt about being selfish, and boldly step forward into living your own life. This book is NOT for you if you're looking for someone to tell you which crystal you should shove in your bra in order to keep "bad vibes" at bay. I will be delivering swift gut punches of real talk and encouraging you to take full responsibility for your journey so if you're here to learn how to "get rid of toxic people" from your life without being willing to take a look at where you yourself are allowing or exhibiting toxicity … you are gonna have a hard time swallowing the nuggets I'm gonna be laying down. BUT if you are ready to have someone talk to you in the 3D, kick your ass, and give you great advice, read on!

By now, you've likely picked up on my inclination for salty language and a very direct and colloquial writing style. This is how I communicate my message and how this entire book is written so if this doesn't resonate with you, it might be best to pop me back on the shelf for someone else, but if you feel my juicy authentic and raw vibes, read on, my friend. We have work to do and I will not be pulling any punches.

I will not mollycoddle you or myself. Compassion, yes ... sympathy, no.

This book is intended to help you use your pain to catalyse your evolution. We are going to shift you from feeling you need to be rescued to finally knowing YOU are a powerful force of nature and you can be empowered in the creation of your life. Let's DO THIS!

CHAPTER 1
HOT MESS EXPRESS – HOW BAD IT GOT

I suppose you don't know what it is when it's happening. The "spiritual awakening."

Looking back I can see so clearly how all this needed to happen in order for me to become the woman I am today and go from being a helpless victim in my own life to a conscious creator badass leading other women to their own empowerment.

Sounds rather grand, doesn't it?

It didn't happen overnight. In fact, as I write this it has been over 10 years since my friend took himself off into the woods and hanged himself in the wee hours of the morning and I got a phone call that sent me spiralling into the deepest, darkest period of my life.

I still remember the phone call.

I had just performed in the opening night of *Educating Rita* and was on a high. I felt like I was unstoppable. You know, those days where it just feels like life has fallen into place and NOTHING can touch you. Glorious!

I was driving through the back lanes on my way to meet another friend to celebrate how well opening night had gone.

My phone rang and I pulled over to answer it … I didn't have Bluetooth back then!

It was a withheld number.

The man on the other end of the phone asked if I was Georgina Noel and I told him I was indeed Miss Noel. I could already feel that something was wrong. I could feel my guts flipping and trying to escape from my body.

"Miss Noel, we need to speak with you, but could you please come to the police station?"

I flatly refused as I was now in complete freeze mode. My body was cold sweating and my heart pounding.

I have revisited this exact fraction of the memory countless times to heal the layers of trauma that occurred. It was like part of me split off and remained trapped in that moment. She was the part of me that held me back for so long – I could feel the trauma in my body for years after, but I didn't know what the feeling of paralysis was. Whenever I would go to DO something big or exciting, I would get the physical sensation of being anchored to the spot. But I'm getting ahead of myself. More on this later.

After a few moments of me sitting wide-eyed and frozen in my car, refusing to budge until I knew what the bloody hell was going on, it clicked …

"Oh my god. It's Fran, isn't it?" He confirmed my worst fears.

Francis was dead.

The next few hours are a bit of blur, but I went to the police station and, whilst sitting in what felt like an interrogation room, I was given a plastic bag, much like one you might put a sandwich in for a packed lunch. In it was the note. Fran's family had said that I should be contacted and invited to read it as I'd been a part of his life leading up to the event.

I remember one thing vividly, as though it was one of those films that is done from the actor's point of view. I remember looking down and seeing my hand holding the envelope and barely being able to make sense of the words I was reading.

My boyfriend at the time was with me and I think he read it to me, but honestly, I can't remember these exact details.

I was numb and, looking back, I think I had completely disassociated from my body because I couldn't process the level of emotion that was coursing through me.

As I read/heard the note, I was waiting for my name to appear and it never did. I remember feeling angry about that.

I know this might sound fucked up, but I was so hurt and confused that he hadn't included me. That I hadn't even crossed his mind in his final moments, or worse still ... I HAD crossed his mind and he had chosen to omit me.

Strange what you feel when your concept of reality has just had a sledgehammer taken to it.

When Fran died, it felt like someone had tipped the contents of my head out on the floor, trod in them, and then squished them back in my head, patted me on the shoulder, and said, "Off y'go." Disorientating, to say the least.

I had never lost someone I was close to before and having a friend die by suicide was the most traumatic event of my life.

So sudden, but also not so sudden when I take into account the years of emotional torment he had been in. It just FELT sudden. It was one of those "that'll never happen to me or someone I know" situations that makes you question the solidity and certainty of everything in your physical reality.

When something like this happens, certainly for me, there was an aspect of feeling that anything I had unconsciously used as a point of safety or anchoring in my life could no longer be relied upon. Anything could be snatched away in the blink of an eye. This outsourcing of safety was something I had always done as I, and possibly you, had never been taught that safety is an internal state of BEING and that we can FEEL safe anytime we choose just by learning how.

Of course, I didn't know that yet and so much fear was activated in my being that day.

I remember standing in the shop the evening after the phone call, whilst on a mission for naan bread (not that the naan is important but I still find it so peculiar that this is what I recall) and I felt like I had been ripped out of the fabric of time and was seeing everything in slow motion. I stood there thinking *How can these people just go about their business? Don't they know he's gone?* I felt as though I'd been split apart from what others saw as real and was now seeing things from a whole new perspective. I was completely disconnected and angry at the world.

The weeks and months after Fran's death were the most painful and confusing of my life.

I kept expecting my phone to ring and to see his number or have him show up at my office door like he used to when he was feeling frail and afraid so that I could soothe his woes with cuddles and cups of tea.

I was unable to function in the world. Nothing seemed important anymore and everyone who was still alive annoyed me.

I became an angry ball of pain and self-destruction. To sleep at night, I had to have all the lights on and the TV on full blast in an attempt to force the voices out of my head with the sheer volume.

I thought the only end to the pain would be to die.

A NOTE ON HEALING BEREAVEMENT: LETTING GO

One of the biggest things I have worked through for myself and with any clients who have experienced a bereavement is the letting go. Once we truly allow ourselves to release the guilt of what we woulda, shoulda, coulda done whilst the person was still alive AND the guilt about us still BEING alive, well, that's when life starts again. That's the moment we get to choose how we are going to move forward and what our life is going to be like from now on.

I was holding on to my grief and guilt because they were the only vaguely tangible things left of Fran and by letting them go, it felt like I was really admitting that he was gone.

By admitting he was gone, I had to then face a world with new truths I wasn't sure I was ready to face. Truths such as the fact that I could not fix everyone. That I needed to deal with my own shit around co-dependency and, most terrifyingly for a lot of us, that I am not in control.

What I didn't know consciously at the time was that, in learning to heal and live again, I was also learning how to release the need for full control in favour of conscious creation, surrender, and the not-so-secret ingredient … trust.

I just want to add at this point, just because you're choosing to LIVE your life because YOU ARE STILL ALIVE does not make you a bad person, and also … they are gone.

What you do now is on you. Whatever you believe about the afterlife, in the case of suicide, it's a fucking bold choice to make and he made it, so it was time for me to forgive myself for not being able to save him and move on with my life.

During this time I was confronted with a core pattern I had run my entire life. I felt a level of guilt and responsibility that I had always carried with me to the point where I didn't know it was something I was able to NOT feel. This event amplified it to the point where it was unavoidable and staring me in the face CONSTANTLY. I felt like it was all my fault. Fran's death, yes, but everything else too. I can now look back down the timeline of my life and prior to Fran's death I can clearly see countless times where I took the blame in an attempt to save someone else's feelings.

I was a people pleaser, but to the max. I would apologise for everything and make myself culpable for even the smallest of errors made by others – particularly if I could see that they were annoyed or frustrated with themselves for said error. I had a very clever way of being able to manipulate the perspective so that I felt I had been the one who'd fucked up. *Why would anyone do this?* I hear you cry. Well, if we are responsible for EVERYTHING, if we are the single human who is to blame for everything, it gives us a strange sense of safety.

It's a control thing.

If it's my fault then there must be a way I can change or control this.

I am a recovering control freak and when I saw this pattern it was huge.

People-pleasing has many facets and I'll speak more on this in Chapter 4, but if you resonate with apologising for others to make them feel better and somehow feeling like you are always in the wrong, constantly treading on eggshells and possibly lingering in procrastination and perfectionism before taking action or making ANY decisions (like … how often do you answer the question "what would you like for dinner?" with "I don't know, what do you fancy?") then YOU, my friend, have a severe case of people-please-itis.

This pattern is so sneaky and insidious that it will be infiltrating every area of your life and the sooner you get it nailed the sooner you'll be free to do whatever the fuck you want and live a life in alignment with your own personal values.

End of rant.

(Worry not, we will look more at this pattern later and I have some nifty strategies and reflections to help you shift out of this and into empowerment. I have got your back!)

TIME TO LOOK THE DEMONS IN THE EYE

I visited Fran's grave only once. In hindsight I think it was a form of wanting to feel the pain of losing him. I was almost addicted to the story and feeling of my pain because it kept him alive, kept me feeling connected to him, and I spent most of my time in numbness so the pain was at least a sensation.

This emotional self-harm had to stop.

That day, after visiting his grave, I looked in the rear-view mirror in my car and I didn't recognise the face looking back at me. I wept. All I saw in those eyes was a deep sadness and a dark emptiness.

I felt hollow.

I honestly did not know how I was ever going to feel okay again.

I remember driving along one day and thinking to myself, *I either go the same way as him and die, or I have to find a way to live.*

And so begins our journey …

CHAPTER 2
I'LL TRY ANYTHING

Months after Fran had died, I started experiencing intense lower back pain. At the first session with my chiropractor she did the intake questions with me, you know the kind of thing … When and where does it hurt? When did it start?

She then asked if I'd experienced anything emotionally traumatic in the last 12 months, to which I replied, "Well, my best friend hanged himself a few months ago. Does that count?" After months of weeping continually and falling to pieces, I was completely numb at this point to any emotional discomfort, walking around in a malaise of nihilistic "meh." Looking back, now I see my body was exhibiting the pain that I was not able to feel emotionally. Anyway … I shan't skip ahead. We will get to that bit shortly …

After revealing what, to any normal human with any ability to actually FEEL, was indeed a rather traumatic event, she responded with, "Ah, yes, that would do it."

She mentioned I might like to try a session of NLP and EFT with her. She told me these sessions were to deal with any underlying emotional causes of physical pain. I didn't really give a fuck, if I'm honest. I just wanted the pain to go away and, at this point, I was so desperate I just told her, "Yeah. Sure. I'll try anything."

I was so completely apathetic by now that I was really just ruling out all options so I could die knowing that I'd tried everything, and so, when I took my own life, I could honestly say, "I tried everything. Nothing worked." Dark, I know, but it's true. Things were bad.

Anyhow, I diligently booked and appeared for my appointment and was met with a very peculiar session indeed.

TAPPEDY-TAP

I didn't have any expectations, but I was obviously hoping that whatever voodoo was about to occur would end this debilitating back pain and I might have some hope of a vaguely normal life if I chose to continue with it.

At this point it's probably worth noting that I had previously attended a few weeks of grief counselling where I got to regale someone with my tales of woe. Here's the problem I had with counselling (before you talk-therapy advocates get your knickers in a knot … I actually trained for four years towards becoming a counsellor a while after I'd regained the will to live so I'm not poo-pooing it entirely; it just, for me and people like us, has its limitations): okay, that said, for me, the problem with counselling was that I am an intelligent woman with what I believe to be a high level of self-awareness and, although this is something I've honed over the years and continue to do so, even back then I wasn't completely unaware of the WHY of my feelings.

And so, repeating the story over and over again in a series of new and exciting ways really didn't do much to quell the ever-expanding desire to just fuck this life off and join my buddy in the ground. I knew I'd had enough of this particular type of therapy when the lady "counselling" me commented that, "He wasn't really very reliable, was he?" Umm ... I get that there's an element of challenging questioning asking in counselling, but come on, dude! Too soon. Too fucking soon.

Anyway, rant over for now, ha ha!

Where counselling left me with a feeling of "Okay, I know WHY I feel this way ... but NOW WHAT?" the experience I had at my first NLP/EFT session with my chiropractor was a completely different story.

She did, of course, ask me to describe how I felt about it and I told her that when he died, "It was like all the lights went out in the world."

The basic premise of the session was this: I brain dump all the feelings and then ... she did some cool fucking magick!

She asked me to say "yes" and then "no" whilst I held my left arm out in front of me. Each time, she pressed lightly on my arm. For YES it held strong. For NO it dropped. It was like I physically COULDN'T keep my arm up and she was barely putting ANY pressure on at all!

She had my attention.

She then asked me to say, "All the lights went out when Fran died," again whilst I held my left arm out in front of me. As I said the phrase she pressed my arm and it stayed firm. She then had me say, "All the lights didn't go out when Fran died," and this time my arm dropped as she gently touched it.

Now I understand that this is a variation of the muscle testing which I use every day! However, back then I'd NEVER been in the presence of anything so fucking COOL and I was immediately captivated.

She had me tap under my eyes whilst repeating the relevant phrase out loud for a few seconds and then we retested. This time the muscle testing results reversed. She explained that my body recognised one phrase as a truth and that we were going in at the root and reprogramming the belief. We were rewiring my brain.

Wide-eyed in wonder and hope. Something was cracking open. I began to feel again. The lights had come back on.

Even writing about this brings a wave of emotion because without this day, I may not be here now, writing this book. Thank you, Sara!

When we are in our darkest of times, we can forget about or reject hope, but when we feel it, we can always choose to lean into it and see where it takes us.

CHAPTER 3
HOLY FUCK – THIS SHIT WORKS

Let's shift gears for a bit and talk about the mind/body connection.

Remember when I mentioned how I have revisited the moment I got the phone call from the police multiple times and healed layers of trauma? I also mentioned how I would experience a physical sensation in my body of being held back or frozen. That is how powerful the mind/body connection is.

This book is by no means a scientific paper nor does it claim to be and so I'm not going to go deep into the workings of the brain, but know this:

Your body stores emotion in its cells (if you want to really dig into this, I recommend reading *Molecules of Emotion* by Candace B. Pert). In simple terms, when we experience trauma, our brain and body take a snapshot of that moment and make decisions based on that information long into our future. I personally have worked with clients who have had severe phobias or allergies in their adult life linked to seemingly unrelated events from their childhood. Once we dissolve the connection between the two, the physical symptoms stop and they go back to their lives.

In Chapter 5 I tell you a story of how EFT helped me heal a physical wound! Bonkers.

When we learn to listen to our bodies rather than bypassing them, we can release so much and ultimately we free ourselves up to experience more of life, and isn't that why you're here on this planet, in this body, reading this book?

If we don't recognise that fear is just the brain's way of protecting us and that it is not always based on REAL information, life can get pretty small pretty quickly.

What does this mean for YOUR life? Well, whenever your soul, higher self, intuition, or whatever you want to call it–that inspired and spontaneous part of you that has all the good, fun ideas – pipes up with a flash of joyful inspiration and within seconds you've talked yourself out of it due to a tightening in your stomach, a flicker of fear in your heart, something that FEELS REAL, and you listen to that feeling instead of the excitement you had at the moment of this idea's conception … that, my friend, is exactly where this kind of energetic and emotional work is going to help you unpack and unlock so much incredible shit in your life!

Imagine having the inspiration, the excitement, and, let's face it, the KNOWING that this thing is for you and then … NOT having the gut wrench, heart flutter of feeling like your bowels might evacuate your body instantly. How fucking EXPANSIVE would your life be if you could deactivate these pre-programmed fear-and-freeze responses in seconds?

Take a moment now to think of a thing you've always wanted to be, do, or have. What happens in your body? Undoubtedly, your brain and internal dialogue got involved too, but BEFORE the story in your head, there was a sensation.

Try it now.

What would happen if that current automatic pattern could be defused and you could just keep leaning in to the feeling of expansion and possibility?

Holy fuck, dude.

This is the shit that really gives me goosebumps.

Here is my first-hand example of how this happened for me IMMEDIATELY after my first session of EFT.

Lemme give you a little context here. One of the main problems I'd been experiencing in my life since Fran died was that every time I looked at someone and perceived them to have even a vague glimmer of sadness in their eyes, I would get this feeling deep in my guts. It felt like TRUTH. I looked at them and I thought *You're going to kill yourself* and it reactivated the panic in my body.

My life had spiralled into a series of triggers that led me to feel completely out of control and so, aside from the blanket numbness that had activated to protect me, I could be, in an instant, gut punched by my own emotions and in utter terror.

I didn't even need something to happen; I was powerfully recreating the trauma over and over again with the power of my mind. Yikes.

It was crippling me emotionally and I was exhausted.

I was isolating myself more and more because being around people was like walking through razor blades.

Okay, enough melodrama, Georgina ... What happened next?

Well, after this first session with Sara, I felt different, but I couldn't quite put my finger on it. Just lighter somehow.

I sat in my car in the carpark and looked into my eyes in the rear-view mirror. I saw a little flicker of life.

What I decided to do next is going to sound a little peculiar, but ... I had to TEST this somehow. I couldn't understand how I could undergo multiple counselling sessions and have people attempt to nurse or pep talk me back into a bundle of joy that they could stand to be around and yet ... one hour with Sara and some weird tapping shit and here I was ... feeling, dare I say ... a little better.

I sat in my car and I TRIED to think about people killing themselves. I know, I know. Twisted. But it was the only way I could know for sure if this voodoo tappy magick had actually worked.

I sat and concentrated, choosing the people to whom I was closest. My boyfriend, close friends, family members. Each one of them I would try to visualise dead and though I could THINK about it ... I couldn't FEEL it. Nothing. It was like the thought entered my head and hit some kind of impenetrable mind trampoline and just bounced straight out again with NO physical or emotional reaction other than my utter RELIEF and sense of wonder.

From that moment I was hooked!

After this first session with Sara I was booking in regularly for everything I could think of! I had spent most of my life, from an early age if I look back, understanding that I KNEW what

I was feeling and often I could trace it back so I understood the bare bones of what an emotional trigger or subconscious pattern/limiting belief was, but I had always carried the question, "So, now what?" What was one to do with all this awareness and understanding?

I had found my answer.

I was like a kid in a sweet shop and training in EFT and NLP were swiftly added to my to-do list. I knew that having people talk their problems round and round in circles was not enough for me and these modalities were the perfect conduit for my intuition to bloom and to really get to help people in the way I always knew I could.

I suppose, looking back, I'd always been drawn to the wounded soldier and wanted to help people, but I'd gone about it in a really unboundaried way because I was just modelling what I'd been taught whilst I was growing up. Co-dependence is NOT the way to support someone who is in pain and now I have bulletproof boundaries which enable me to take care of my heart whilst also being able to support, motivate, and inspire others to heal their own lives and step up into their higher purpose.

CHAPTER 4
RELEASING THE PEOPLE PLEASER BY OWNING YOUR TRIGGERS

Co-dependency has many guises, one of which is the need to ask for permission or the need for others to acknowledge our way as THE way. I have also had co-dependency show up as a need for approval.

One of the most common ways to identify if you have people-please-itis is by asking yourself if you put the needs of others before your own in ANY way. No matter how small, this is a sneaky little fucker and shows up everywhere if not plucked out at the root and reframed.

The best way to illustrate this is to tell you a little about my journey with money.

I used to think that the only way I would ever be truly happy was to make sure everyone around me was happy first. I now see how that was a weird way of me needing other people's permission to be okay. Permission and releasing the need for it has been another juicy knot I got to untie for myself.

I started to notice it when I began my money mindset and wealth consciousness journey in 2016. I started making a lot of money in my business and I had a fun little ritual of, after securing a big sale, going to my favourite clothes shop and just buying anything I wanted. I would take as many things as I could into the changing room, try them all on, and buy everything that made me feel and look good.

One day I was so in flow that I walked into a shop and the lady behind the counter handed me an envelope with £2k cash in it and told me she wanted to work with me and hadn't got round to booking in online so would I accept cash?! I mean ... WTF?!

Anyway, things were going great and I went to my fave shop to seal in the magick and celebrate. When I got home, I bounced into the living room totally high on the crazy synchronicities I had experienced and my boyfriend looked concerned. "Shouldn't you be saving some money?" Oof. I took that like a punch to the guts!

How fucking dare he tell me what to do with MY money? I worked hard for this and had been hustling away for YEARS to get to this point and now he was telling me I shouldn't be spending; nay, that I was being IRRESPONSIBLE ... How VERY dare he?

Okay ... breathe, Noel, breathe. He had a point and let's be honest, if he said anything like that to me today it wouldn't even touch the sides. Although he wouldn't say that now because I have healed that shit and <u>I no longer project out that vibration. It's all an inside job, bishes!</u>

So, I lost my shit at him and then went into another guilt-and-shame spiral. Let's look back at my assumption from his one little comment.

He at NO point said that I was being irresponsible and even if he had, if it doesn't ring true for me in my own beliefs about myself, it wouldn't have triggered the fuck out of me!

It was I who'd interpreted his words to mean I was being irresponsible because part of me felt that I was. My little spending sprees were completely harmless and a great way to keep myself elevated in my money vibes which meant more money just kept coming, but in that moment I sabotaged my own vibration with going down the rabbit hole and telling myself a story of how I just spend and I should be more grown up with my finances and blah and blah and blah.

You see … unless we are holding a belief about ourselves, we can't be penetrated in this way. It was NOT his fault that I felt how I felt. That was all me.

My need for him to get on board with my decision on what to do with my money came from me needing his approval and permission.

When we are little kids, we usually don't have our own source of income outside of the adults in our life. I didn't get given pocket money. I remember asking for it once because I heard some kids at school talking about it. My mum didn't see the point because she said I could just ask her for the thing and then she would buy it for me. Sounds ideal, right?

However, it gave me a pattern of feeling that I needed permission or that I required someone else to sign off on what I wanted in order to receive it. Me asking for pocket money was about having a little something that was mine and that could be spent on whatever I wanted.

I was always encouraged to save as a kid. In fact, my birthday and Christmas money would go straight in my savings and I never even thought of it as money that belonged to me until I got into my teens and I remember buying a shirt with some birthday money. I was quizzed on said shirt and the validity or necessity of its purchase. In order to soften the blow, I lied and told my mum and dad it was only about £20. It ended up being £45 but I was so in love with that purple-and-orange tie-dyed blouse (holy fuck … what was I thinking, ha ha! Let's just blame the early nineties and go about our day, shall we!!). I bought the blouse and felt SO GUILTY that I immediately hid it from my parents. I was so anxious I would get found out for spending so much without their approval.

And so, ladies and gentlemen of the jury, now we can clearly see where the reaction came from. It came from a 13-year-old me and I was 34 when I had this first big business year, so maybe it was time to shift out of that pattern and get my shit in order.

My need to stay within the boundaries and rules created by other people in order to keep myself safe by keeping them happy has really been one of my biggest identity shifts.

When you can master your ability to be in your sovereignty and own your decisions and desires, you will set yourself free.

OKAY, NOEL, BUT HOW DO I MASTER MY SOVEREIGNTY?!

The best tip I can give you here is to get super honest with yourself about who you are actively holding on to in your life. Who do you feel you would completely dissolve without?

Now ask yourself how much of what you ALLOW yourself to be, do, and have is connected with your need to keep them in your life versus what YOU want from a place of your innermost desires?

I didn't say this would be a walk in the park, but getting down and dirty with your own desires is a big part of what will reconnect with an innate sense of aliveness and purpose.

Being driven by what we want is completely different from creating goals and a life plan based on what we think other people want of us, being so afraid to lose somebody or to move us away from what we think will hurt.

When you let what YOU want lead the way, you're gonna surprise yourself at how easy and fun life gets to be if you let it!

CHAPTER 5
AND THEN I GOT STABBED

Like, for reals. With a carving knife. Dramatic, right?!

This is the story of a series of unfortunate events involving me being needy, unboundaried, having low self-worth, and seeking outside approval.

It is also the story of how I got stabbed with a carving knife during a live performance of Hamlet.

BOUNDARIES AND SELF-RESPONSIBILITY

I was so desperate to fit in and be accepted that, even when I felt VERY uncomfortable about the use of real carving knives and running towards one another (I am eye rolling at myself over here), I STILL did the play.

Lemme get this straight. Today, if this same situation happened I would raise an eyebrow at the director and tell him to go fuck himself, but back then, I was a little more meek when it came to things like this and, although I've always been outspoken and bolshy, I was well versed in being the good girl and not wanting to look like the one who "wouldn't join in" or go along with the authority figure's demands. I also outsourced my safety to others and when I was informed that everyone was excited about the prospect of actual BLADES being run around the set, I felt like I was being a killjoy wimpy pants and should just man the fuck up.

Oh, Georgina. You did pay handsomely for this one.

In rehearsals we, the cast, were directed to stand in two lines facing each other, each of us holding a carving knife blade pointed out in front of us. We were strategically scattered so that when we ran towards each other – yes, you read that correctly – we would skim past each other but with enough room in between each of us that we would not slice each other in half.

At least, that was the plan.

It was terrifying and I felt very on edge about it, but the whole rest of the cast were so fucking pumped about it that I ignored my intuition and opted for being a team player.

Here's the juicy twist ...

During the live performance, the director changed things. He would walk over to a member of the cast and whisper a new stage direction to them, and this meant that as performers, we, just like the audience, had no idea what was coming next ... Ay caramba.

Yes, it makes for a certain visceral flair and crackle of energy in the air, but it also made for 18 stitches in my arm and around three months of painkillers, surgery, and pain.

As the performance went on I was convinced the director would not give the cue for the knife running. I thought *Yeah, he just did that so we are all on edge and have this electric energy during performance and there's no way we are going to have to actually DO the knife running.*

I was wrong.

Not only did we get the cue, but due to his really exciting directing style (eye roll) there was now a prop directly in my path. I was wearing a huge petticoat and corset so there was no way for me to leap over the fucking thing. I had to dodge it by swerving round it. The person opposite me did not swerve to compensate and so …

Slicey, slicey.

The knife ripped through the flesh of my left elbow.

I felt what I can only describe as someone tugging on the sleeve of your jumper. My brain recognised this as a bad sign, dropped my knife, grabbed the wound, and ran over to the director to whom I calmly stated, "I have just been stabbed so I need to go to the hospital." I left the auditorium and had my friend call me an ambulance and three more of my fabulous friends applauded and cheered "Brava" as I got carted away to the hospital. It really was quite the performance.

The play continued, in case you were wondering. The audience thought I was just an incredible actor and that it was part of the show! That's how fucking nuts that play was!

THE BLAME GAME

I'm not proud to admit it, but I went deep into blame on this one. I was so hurt that nobody had stood up for me. No one had protected me. Nobody had stopped the play. I was victiming hard. Even to the point where I had lawyers attempt to sue the director. The case wouldn't stick. Back then I felt so disempowered and out of control of my life that I just needed to do something. I needed someone to be culpable for what had happened. Surely things like this can't just happen?

At this point, it might be worth you reflecting on where you are blaming others for the shit that's happened in your life. Back when this happened, I was running a pattern of needing to be rescued in order to feel loved and safe. I didn't even understand the concept of resourcing safety from within. I had always needed to be taken care of to some extent.

Here's the thing about a belief like that. If love and safety = being rescued, I will also be playing that out in how I show others I love them. I automatically felt the urge to rescue people I love and if they didn't need rescuing, I felt like I was no use to them. What a mess.

This probably comes from when I was a little kid. I was the baby – there's 13 and 15 years between my sisters and I (yes, there're more of us!) – and so I was kinda the happy surprise and was treated as such.

I was wrapped in cotton wool my entire childhood, protected from EVERYTHING, and I ended up running a lot of beliefs around the world being a dangerous place and that my life purpose was just to STAY ALIVE and cling on to anything and anyone that made me feel safe.

Look, my mum is an amazing woman and now I have a relationship with her where I have actually thanked her for modelling to me some awesome traits. She is incredibly kind and generous, for example, but from childhood I remember her fear and anxiety and an almost desperate feeling of always being unsafe was deeply palpable. If you're reading this – love you, Mum!

So, even though I was loved by way of "She is precious. Keep her alive!" which might sound like a good thing, I always had this inner sadness. My mum even told me about a time when I was just a tiny person after one of my grandparents had died. I wouldn't get out of the car and when she tried to coax me out, I said, "Nobody else is going to die, are they?" Yikes. Even at an early age I was a sensitive little soul and picked up on the energy of the household.

Looking back, one of the reasons my mum likely went in so hard on the protection vibe was that she is also very sensitive and I think she recognised it in me and was trying to protect me from my own emotions, but as we know, that is not possible.

My ability to perceive energy and emotions was overwhelming when I was a little kid and I have another memory where I was sitting on the stairs at my childhood home and I just remember the feeling. It is what adult me would refer to as a feeling of depression or emptiness. I was crying, what felt like continually, and this particular memory is of when a member of my family came up the stairs to appease me, and now I understand she was likely worried about me and not feeling sure how to deal with this tiny person displaying such dark emotions, but back then I felt dismissed and as though I should just suck it up, but … I didn't know how.

I see this a lot. Beautiful souls who have felt punished for their ability to feel deeply and, if that is you, I just want to take this opportunity to say that these traits are a GIFT. If you implement the tools in this book you CAN take back control of your emotions and learn to use your intuition to support you and those around you on your terms, rather than feeling like you're the universe's puppet. What you are is, in fact, an incredible human with a huge capacity for love and joy and when you learn to implement and uphold solid boundaries, you will fall in love with your sensitivity to energy and emotions.

Okay, preach mode disengaged. Let's get back to the main story.

During the healing process of the stabbing injury I got to heal some of these deep co-dependency, self-worth, and safety wounds which have been life changing to this day. So, every cloud …

IT'S NOT HEALING

After a few weeks of devouring painkillers I had my stitches removed and the skin had died. It was black. Oh, I should probably have warned you this chapter might get a bit gross. Ha ha!

The skin had no feeling and was literally dead. If I could insert a vomit face emoji here, I would.

I found out I had to get a debridement which is basically where they put you under general anaesthetic and cut the dead flesh away. They then scoop out all the infection (I may actually vom myself whilst describing this!) and leave you with an open wound which needs constant tending.

The injury was on my left elbow so I could not bend my arm.

It was a pretty shitty time, to be honest.

It got infected AGAIN and there was talk of me needing a skin graft, which would mean that I would have another open wound on my ass cheek and an unsightly graft site on my arm.

I'm telling you all this because my aim is for you to understand that I was doing everything right. I was resting, taking my pills, going for regular wound cleaning and redressing appointments, keeping the site of the injury dry … I was following all the rules and still this fucking wound would not heal.

Nobody could tell me why this kept happening.

Amidst this really pleasant experience I had booked in to see Sara for another session of magic tapping and my intention was to deal with my sugar addiction because food and I have a long history … Maybe that'll be book number two!

Anyway, I showed up to my appointment and was still unable to bend or move my arm, was in constant pain, and yet I still wanted to work on weight loss.

It hadn't even occurred to me that we could tap for healing the fucking stab wound!! WTF?!

As I entered the room, Sara looked down at my bandaged arm and asked me about it. I regaled her with the tale and then set about my story of weight gain and sugar addiction. She asked if I'd mind doing a few clearing statements around the arm injury.

I will confess, I thought this was an epic waste of my time and money, but I did it anyway because … people pleaser. Only this time, my need to please others paid off in my favour!

She asked me to describe the events leading up to and after the stabbing. As I began telling her the story I felt the AHA moment land.

You know that feeling. The lightbulb moment. I love a good lightbulb moment!!

I got stabbed on the Friday night and my boyfriend at the time came with me to the hospital, took me back to his flat, and looked after me for two solid days. We actually had a lovely time together despite the hole in my appendage.

We did "coupley things."

Now look, I'm not gonna go deep into our relationship right now, but what is relevant here is that this was the FIRST time we had spent an entire weekend together in the two years of our relationship.

It was on this day I truly learnt the meaning of secondary gain or "the reason for keeping the problem."

For a long time I had read about and understood this idea that we create our own reality and that we call events, people, and things to us because of how we perceive the world. I got it on an intellectual level, but wasn't actively living that as my truth and it was this experience that really brought this lesson home for me.

I really "got it" this time.

In the moment of the stabbing trauma my body and brain had decided that I had to remain injured and in pain in order to receive love.

Looking back, I can see the seed of this pattern was also sown in childhood when my mother would tend to me so attentively and I would receive treats and all the attention whenever I was even slightly sick. This is often the case with trauma. The initial pattern and beliefs are planted in early childhood and then later in life a series of what can even be smaller traumas (although, admittedly, getting stabbed in front of an audience is rather a big trauma) will trigger the secondary trauma and you'll end up with what was once a whisper from within being a bit more SHOUTY and SORT THIS THE FUCK OUT!!!

Can you see anywhere in your own life where you have locked in negative or limiting beliefs in a moment of severe trauma?

What are the patterns that seem to repeat for you that can be traced back to the early years of your life?

Within three days of that EFT session, the wound started to heal over.

Mind officially blown.

YOU GET WHAT YOU BELIEVE YOU DESERVE

I know it might not be the easiest pill to swallow, but you are creating everything you see in your life right now and everything that has happened to you.

When we allow ourselves to connect the dots we can either get mad about it and beat ourselves up or push blame on to other people, our upbringing, current circumstances, OR we can take ownership of it and allow ourselves to feel the awakening as a moment of clarity and empowerment.

Deciding to OWN your shit and take radical self-responsibility for the life you're living is exactly where things will begin to turn around for you and all you have to do is choose to feel empowered by this concept rather than victimised.

We have established at this point that we all love to be in control in our own way and what better way to nurture our inner control freak than to say, "Hey, dude, I am literally in control of everything I call in to my life and how I respond to it." BOOM!

Try it now. Where in your life are you feeling out of control and like there is chaos? Where are you feeling you need someone else to rescue you? Before you spiral into all the reasons why it is not your fault, take a moment and ask yourself from a space of curiosity, "How did I create this? How is this serving me?"

"Where am I feeling I need someone else to change so that I can be happy?" This is a biggie. When we start living our lives from a place of understanding that WE are choosing how we respond, react, and feel about things, we get to change everything! Argh! It's amazing!

This book could end right here and if you implement this your life will change forever.

But I got more to say, so let's continue.

CHAPTER 6
IT ALL STARTS WITH YOU

Part of my story is the bit where I decided I no longer wanted to work a full-time job doing things that had begun to feel like I was killing time and not really making an impact on the world.

I had a small income at the time as I was working for an arts charity, but I knew I had to start investing in retraining and nurturing this part of me that so desperately wanted to help people.

The thing I loved most about starting this journey was that I also got to work on my own shit!

Even in the counselling course we got weekly journalling homework where we were encouraged to reflect on the events of the week using the tools we were learning, and I found it fascinating. I'd always been what my mum called a "deep thinker" (as an aside, once she told me in exasperation, "Oh, Georgina, you're too deep for me," and I remember taking that on as a truth for everyone. My depth of thought and intensity have ended up being some of the qualities that have been most helpful in my purpose work, so just remember that you're never too much of anything – you're exactly the right amount of everything to be the perfect YOU).

Anyway, I took this opportunity to plumb my own depths and found myself quite fascinating. All these patterns and thoughts that I had on autopilot had created this kind of web in which I was living my life and now I could see how just changing the way I see a situation or what thought I decide is true could alter my reality.

Things were getting interesting!

I became addicted to this self-development lark and did a number of courses. I began to notice something that unsettled me. Not everyone had my same passion for unlocking their own shit. There seemed to be a few people on each course that wanted to help others, without ever really looking at themselves. This to me seems problematic. If we are not willing to get honest with ourselves about our own perceptions and limitations, how are we ever to see clearly into the soul or truth of another?

I just knew that if someone was pissing me off, then it's more about me than them.

This was the beginning of me implementing mirror theory, though I had no idea that was even a thing back then.

In brief, mirror theory is a way of using what we see and experience in the world as a reflection of what exists in us. For example, if I see your beauty, I can only see it in you because it also exists in me. However, if I see pain or sadness in you, the likelihood is that I am actually seeing a projection of my own pain.

One of the examples I give during my EFT practitioner trainings is when you want to go and hug someone. You see them, perceive them as sad or "in need of a hug," but often that hug is more for you than for them. If we do not go about "cleaning our mirror" and getting clearer and clearer on our own subconscious patterns and belief systems it can be hard for us to ever see anyone clearly because we are unconsciously projecting. When you use mirror theory it can be a bit of a head fuck to start with, but if you go in with a view to being curious and learning more about yourself with the purpose of understanding how you can be a more balanced and open human, it is incredibly freeing!

At first I judged the fuck out of these people on the courses. Ha ha! I would look at them and perceive them to be whinging about shit that I could see would be easy to change and it irritated me. They were blaming the world for their problems and that made me want to drop kick them. However, when I started to own my shit and realise that ANY judgements we have of others are all about us, things got juicy!

It was another lightbulb moment of, "Fuuuuck. Where am I projecting out and blaming others for how I feel or what has happened to me?" It was a reality check and although some of them still irritated me, I started to use it to my advantage and learn more about how I could heal.

When I could see the projections in people on these programs, I became a curious observer and rather than taking on the judgements I decided to learn. I began watching and witnessing their backgrounds, having empathy for them, but realising they are just recreating the same things over and over again in their lives.

Some would be embodying their victim whilst feeling powerless against the bullies in their past from childhood through their adult life and yet … they were also a bully in their own way. They couldn't see where they were the perpetrator. This led me into even deeper self-reflection and I began asking myself shadow questions like, "Where am I not owning my inner bully? Where am I allowing myself to feel victimised because I'm afraid of being PERCEIVED as a bully?" So much juice in these kinds of questions – give it a go!

On these courses I witnessed a lot of blame and projecting out.

What really got my goat about this was when people would hold on so tight to needing everything to be someone else's fault and some terrible shit had happened to these people – myself included. Here is my #realtalk on this:

Okay, you feel that you were wronged. Are you going to keep letting that person hurt you even though they likely no longer even feature in your day-to-day life? Are you going to CONTINUE ALLOWING your abuser, ex-partner, parents, childhood bully to control how you feel about yourself and your ability to create an EPIC life for yourself? NO? Good. So, it's time to step the fuck up and do whatever it takes to release all that trapped emotion. There are a number of resources to help you with this that you can access listed at the back of this book.

When you are trapped in a cycle of thinking and feeling that someone else is to blame for how YOU feel, you'll never truly be happy. So why on earth would we hold on to all this crap? What's the reason for keeping the problem here?

Well, if it's not our responsibility we don't have to do the scary work of transformation which could mean outgrowing people or circumstances in which we have become ensconced. I know how scary this can be. Trust me! Not wanting to "leave people behind" was one of the BIGGEST things that kept me in self-sabotage until I realised that the more inner work I did on myself, the better fit the new people were that I was attracting and some of the people from the previous "life" stepped up and felt inspired by my growth so they actually grew too!

If someone can only love you or feel safe with you when you are stuck and in pain that is a reflection of their lack of ability to resource safety from within themselves and you don't need that shit weighing you down. The people who are meant to continue on with you will raise their fucking game and the rest will fall away, but rest assured there are plenty of other people out there who are equally as obsessed with self-development as you and you WILL find them if you just stay true to your journey, trust, and keep moving forward.

Plus, my desire to bring the world and his dog on my journey with me was partly based in my own fear that I would end up alone and as you will find out during this book, the opposite is actually true. Hurrah!

CHAPTER 7
SO, YOU'VE GOT A THING FOR BAD BOYS

For as long as I can remember, I have been a little obsessed with darkness. Even as a kid, I always wanted the bad guys to win; I identified with the villain compared to the princess, because I thought they were misunderstood. I felt sorry for them in a way.

From a young age, I wanted people to be accepted and understood. To me, the way that the goodie would end up vilifying and being mean to the baddies made them even WORSE than the original villains!

Learning about and implementing shadow work helped me to understand why I identified with them in this way.

Anytime we reject a quality or have an adverse reaction to someone, it's because we are not owning our shadow.

So, let's say you don't like bullies. Here are some things to ponder:

Where in my life am I being a bully?

Where am I persecuting others or myself?

What does my reaction to the bully tell me about my own ability to be boundaried and say no?

There are MANY ways we could dig into this but there's some food for thought.

ANYTIME we make a sweeping generalisation about someone based on our projections, we are blind to how they might be reflecting back to us traits which we have not admitted to ourselves that live within us.

This polarising – bully bad; victim good – means that we can overcorrect and play the victim because we are so inherently fearful of becoming, or even worse, being PERCEIVED as a bully by others.

Oh, what a tangled web we weave.

Lemme give you an example from my own experience to take the sting out of it!

In past romantic relationships I was very willing to play the victim, and not really look at the shadow. At first glance, I always went for people who were emotionally manipulative, withholding in some way. It was only when I distanced myself from them that I realised I had been playing into the manipulation which is, in itself, a form of manipulation! "Poor me" bullshit – eurgh!

Here's an unpopular nugget but it's how I see the world, so buckle up, we are going IN!

The narcissist can only be the narcissist if there is someone willing to play into the victim role, otherwise they're just an asshole.

When we understand that we are, on some level, willingly playing into that role we once again take back control of our brains and hearts and get to do some self-reflection, and more specifically in this case, some shadow integration.

My ex, though incredibly handsome and charming, was emotionally constipated. I was, therefore, besotted. Completely obsessed with him.

I would show up at his house, let myself in, and do his washing up and leave freshly baked cookies. At the time I thought it was really nice and helpful, but it was actually just manipulative.

I knew on a subconscious level that I was never going to get what I wanted from him and so he was a safe place for me to pour my love and adoration without any danger of it being fully reciprocated.

If he had given me the storybook Prince Charming kinda love, I would have fucked it up in another way because I wasn't ready for what I said and thought I wanted.

I was in no way ready to receive love or a genuine heart connection at that time in my life.

I was TERRIFIED of loss. I thought anything good could be ripped from me at a moment's notice. I remember one of my early business coaches commenting on how I always seemed to be "waiting for the other shoe to drop." I could never just enjoy something. I was always bracing for when the tide would turn and everything would turn to shit. Again, this is likely the product of being brought up surrounded by a lot of fear and anxiety, but at some point you have to stop blaming your parents and do the fucking healing work. Am I right?

I chose a man so preoccupied with his own life struggles and trauma (of which he did have plenty) that he didn't have the emotional capacity to give me more and so I got to play out my story of "Even when I give my everything, the man I want doesn't want me!" Sheesh.

Once again, I was determined to prove to myself that I had no control over my life, that I was worthless and a victim, but then the stabbing happened and I learnt about how I'd been effectively giving away my power because the thought of actually taking responsibility for my life and my choices had felt like it was too big for me. I felt like I was still a child in some ways. Needing to be rescued and shown how to live.

My relationship with this man was so rich in learning, and with hindsight I see how it was totally necessary for us both.

So how did I integrate the shadowy shit, in this case, the victim? Through more EFT and self-exploration I began to really get what this shadow shit was about. I began admitting my deep, dark truths. I started working with a shadow animal: I would visualise a shark tearing people apart and really fucking them up. I began Muay Thai and learned to channel my aggression and anger in a positive way. As women in particular, we are taught that anger, violence, and rage are bad things and so we never truly get to express them, and even less likely is it that we would be witnessed, held, and loved in our fullest expression of these emotions!

Anyway, back to the topic at hand, Georgina.

My integration of the victim came after I used various shadow integration practices, such as the shadow animal and journalling all the dark shit out of my head without judgement – that's the key here … ZERO JUDGEMENT.

Seeing the contents of your brain in this way is confronting, but so bloody cathartic! When I let myself FEEL the extremes of myself, I begin to realise that I would never really do any of the things my darkest thoughts would've had me believe, but in honouring them through journalling, for example, I was giving them an outlet and I was no longer afraid of those thoughts. Bringing them into the light defused the fear.

After my last relationship I drew a line in the goddamn sand. I would NEVER treat myself that way again and I would never be the victim. I was gonna be an independent woman! Then I met my current partner – poor sod! He met me when I was being initiated into my own fire and standing up for what I wanted.

It took a while, but eventually I found that by rejecting the victim completely, I became a tyrant and, not ironically, a victim, but in a whole new way.

It was only when I gave myself permission to love that needy little kid inside of me, the one who just wanted to be held and loved with all her imperfections and vulnerability, did I truly understand that both the victim and the tyrant are necessary and safe when I don't force one of them out!

The tyrant has some incredibly powerful qualities for me. She owns her NO and has kick-ass boundaries, she puts her needs and energy as a priority, and doesn't take any shit. The victim understands the softer, squishier bit of me and others and so she can help me empathise and be compassionate.

Y'see! ALL of these qualities are SO valuable and help to lead an empowered life, but we must be willing to own the fact that sometimes we would quite like to punch someone in the face for being a dick whilst simultaneously questioning the dick within.

FRIENDING IS HARD! THE VULNERABILITY OF HEART CONNECTION

Well, now you know how I found romantic relationships, let's talk about friendship. If you're anything like me, which if you've made it this far into this book, likelihood is you're vibing with what I'm puttin' down so I'm gonna make the bold assumption that you are a bit like me. You lucky fucker!

You've likely felt completely fucked over by friendships and closed off your heart to true soulmate friends. I didn't even believe this was a real-life thing until February 2019 when I met two women who shifted my whole perspective on friendship and holy mama, how things have changed!

But before I tell you about these badasses, let's go back.

Ay caramba. This has been another journey and a half!

OWNING THE DARKNESS

Now feels like a good time to tell you a little bit more about the nature of my relationship with my friend Fran and how this impacted my ability to allow people into my heart.

I am about to share with you some dark truths about how my brain worked and forgiving myself for this has been a huge part of my healing process, so remember as you read that wherever you are harbouring patterns or thoughts that make you feel like a "bad person" or if you have things it is hard to admit to yourself because of self-judgement or fear of what others would think, you were doing the best you could with resources you had at the time and that now you get to heal, grow, and move forward with a new perspective and more empowered mindset.

Okay, so, we had dated for a while when I was about 19 and I was besotted with him. He was the most beautiful man I'd ever seen and I couldn't believe that HE wanted ME. I had an array of incredibly beautiful friends … In my mind, I was the funny one. He could've had his pick of any number of beauties, and yet he chose me. So, yeah, you could say I had some self-esteem issues, but I didn't have the first drop of awareness around that yet. At that age I honestly believed all the bullshit my brain told me.

You're fat, ugly, weird, and broken … pretty much that on repeat. I had some really vicious self-talk. It's so interesting to write about this now because I am so far from that these days. Even if my brain has a moment of "going to town on me" I am always witnessing it and able to just let it play itself out and find a way of reframing it. I also allow myself to actually FEEL my emotions these days.

I had always been very good at speaking about and articulating emotions, but I didn't really start to feel them until I went through The Spiral in 2018. Whew! That was a ride! But I'll come back to that later.

For now, let's get back to the most beautiful man who ever lived and how his attention validated the living fuck out of me.

We never got serious, Fran and I, but he would often call me his soulmate and I found out after his death that his family had always hoped and expected us to end up together. The events leading up to his death were complicated in terms of our relationship. I was in an on-again-off-again relationship with my now ex and Fran, in his wounded and vulnerable state, provided a place for me to receive adoration. Eurgh. As I write that I can feel my guts turning. I knew what I was doing, but I felt powerless to my own lack of self-worth. I didn't feel special in my romantic relationship and so I was outsourcing my need to feel special to Fran and, even though it was from a very wounded place, I could feel how much he needed me and at the time, I was running a very deeply ingrained pattern that NEED = LOVE. We were playing out our own private little co-dependent bubble and neither of us had the presence of mind to stop it.

As I'm writing this I feel my mind acknowledging judgement coming up around how manipulative I seem when I look back on this. Today I know that I get to take charge of how I feel and I am SO aware of any co-dependency shit that comes up. I mean, I'm not perfect, but I definitely notice it these days when it pops up and I have been working through a lot of this stuff which I will share with you before the end of this chapter, but because of my awareness NOW it can be all too easy to judge myself for what I did when I actually DIDN'T understand I could walk away, set boundaries, etc. I was AFRAID to set boundaries in case he didn't want me anymore and then I'd have to face the stark reality that I was, in my mind, less than ordinary.

I was afraid to walk away in case he killed himself and it was all my fault.

I was afraid to set the record straight and I dangled the false hope of us uniting through my actions, if not through my words. I thought I loved this man, but really it was what he reflected back to me that I loved.

These imaginary consequences I concocted in all my relationships and it meant that I was so desperate to keep people in favour, I would contort myself into whatever flavour of human I felt they desired. I've always been an intuitive little fucker and I used it against myself back then in order to "become" what others needed me to be.

Oof, what a mindfuck!

That's part of co-dependency though. Have you ever felt like that about someone? It's like you need them to fill the void in your heart and soul. They are a distraction from the emptiness that lies beneath the surface, almost like an addiction sometimes.

Here is what I have learned and this is what helped me turn this shit around, set myself free, and call in TRUE soulmate friends and conscious connections.

I now ask myself:

What is this person reflecting back to me?

How do they "make me feel" and where am I not allowing myself to feel that without needing external validation or stimuli?

What unowned part of myself am I seeing/judging here?

For example, Fran made me feel special and valuable. He made me feel needed, which I equated with love and safety. That 25-year-old me did NOT feel any of those things inside, but longed to so desperately and would do whatever it took to get and keep them.

Lemme just say here that if you're sitting there beating yourself up for all the shit that is coming up for you, all the times you could've "done better," just remember that forgiving yourself and understanding that part of living life with full self-responsibility is that we are responsible for the part WE played, but the other people in our lives are also responsible for THEIR actions and choices. This is the bit people often forget. Whether the people around choose to own their shit is also not your responsibility. So, take a breath and remember you are a good human and you are on a journey. Nobody needs you to be perfect or you may as well sprout wings and ascend already!

Whenever we outsource our sense of self-worth or safety to another human or ANYTHING outside of ourselves, we are setting ourselves up to fall flat on our ass because nobody can ever give us everything we need apart from ourselves. I'm not saying you need to isolate yourself and be totally alone and never depend on anyone ever again; in fact, I went so far that way after I started noticing my co-dependent streak that I shut my heart almost entirely and it was quite painful crowbarring it open again, but I often operate that way. I will be all in on one way of being, notice it is unhealthy, and then pendulum swing all the way over to the other side, find out why THAT is also fucked up, and then I find my happy balance in the middle. It's a ride! Ha ha!

Today, I have incredible friends with whom I can be SO open and honest about triggers or co-dependency shit that I have gone a long way to healing it. Where I once felt powerless in relationships, I now understand that anything I see or feel is my shit and with the right people, I can own that shit and they will openly and consciously help me through it from a place of non-judgement and we trust each other to take full self-responsibility for owning our triggers and bring them to the table. This leads to a level of open communication I had never even dreamed could be real … but it is and I am so fucking grateful.

A part of the story with Fran is that my then-boyfriend and I had split up again and it was Fran's birthday so a group of us went out to celebrate. He had been seeming so much better for a few days. He did seem a little angry at times, but I think we were all just SO glad he had stopped obsessively talking about his suicidal thoughts that we chose to be blind to the warning signs that this was a shadow version of the man we all knew and loved.

I went back to his apartment after and things got heated. We kissed and I stayed over. He wanted to have sex and as soon as we lay down together I could feel his energy and it was dark. My intuition kicked me from inside and made me stop. I explained that it wasn't that I didn't want him, it was just that I didn't want it to happen like this. It was like my higher self shook me and woke me the fuck up. I could finally see clearly and I knew that if this happened I would be trapped. I didn't want him to ONLY want me when he was sick. The reality was, he only ever contacted me when he was depressed and needed someone to hold his pain. I told him, when he was feeling better, that if he still wanted this, we would go for it and live happily ever after, but that this was not the time. He was angry or maybe just frustrated with the situation, me, himself. The truth is, I will never know what was really happening for him at that moment. We fell asleep and I left the next morning for a show rehearsal.

He wouldn't answer my texts all day and when I spoke to him on the phone that night we had an argument and I was desperately trying to get him to forgive me. He was so despondent. I couldn't get him to say he loved me. He always told me he loved me, but not that night. He numbed out to me, went cold, and I was heartbroken and panicking.

I tried to call him several times after that and he wouldn't answer his phone. Desperate to make sure he didn't "do anything silly," I called his sister and she called him to check in.

The next day was opening night of my show. That was the night he died.

Our final conversation was a fucking disaster and I have had to live with that every day since. I felt so much guilt and shame. I genuinely thought that his death was my fault.

SELF-RESPONSIBILITY VS "IT'S ALL MY FAULT"

This was a stark lesson in self-responsibility versus the "It's all my fault" default mindset I spoke about in Chapter 1. Owning your vibration and your part in the creation of your world is not the same as believing everything is your fault.

Believing everything is your fault is just that – a belief. It's not real. Self-responsibility is a way of being in the world and a conscious decision to see yourself as the point of attraction in your life where you get to CHOOSE how you show up in the world on all levels: physically, emotionally, energetically.

That felt like an important distinction to make.

Okay, continuing forth … Let's go!

HOW TO PRISE OPEN YOUR COLD, DEAD HEART

I mentioned that I pendulum swung from "let me help you, I am your saviour and will protect you from your own feelings" to shutting myself down after Fran's death. I was protecting myself and it can happen after a bereavement or a break-up. That feeling that things could all be ripped away in an instant. Cultivating my inner sense of safety was a vital part of healing this pattern.

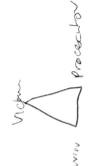

The more stuff, success, love I got, the more afraid I was that I would lose it and so I would sabotage my own success and happiness because if I fucked it up at least I was in control.

Yowzers.

It can be super vulnerable to let people in and actually FEEL them and let them feel and see you. The thought that I might love someone and then lose them kept me from connection with people for years. I knew I had to start healing my heart and so I went for Craniosacral with an amazing lady I'd met on the counselling course. She spoke to my body and I felt so safe in her energy that I allowed my heart to start cracking open.

I'm not going to bullshit you and say that I had one session and suddenly love rushed into my veins and I felt safe to spread seeds of joyous soul connection far and wide, because that would be a big fat lie. I would say, this part of my process has taken at least three years. Healing my heart and being able to love myself and others has really been an ongoing thing and once again, I have The Spiral to thank for speeding this journey up. That mother fucker cracks you open like no process I have ever experienced before.

In January of 2020 I went through The Spiral for a third time and I went in with the intention of activating and opening my heart. I will tell you more about The Spiral in a moment, but for now I want to share with you my experience of the vulnerability and beauty of accessing our heart.

I am not sure I ever felt safe being loved. I never really trusted it. I was waiting for the moment it would change or be withheld. Love came with strings and expectation attached.

Meeting the people in The Spiral community and finding my tribe within the tribe has been a gentle journey of being held, witnessed, and supported through my shadows, reflections, and projections. My two closest and most beautiful friends from that community had been party to my continual unfolding and I to them.

No co-dependency. No expectation. Just pure love, respect, and soul connection. Even a year ago I didn't think it was possible for me, but here I am exploring sisterhood and actually enjoying it!

When we have experienced hurt and unbalanced relationships, it is quite normal for us to be protective of our heart, but here's the thing: If we are love, if we are able to embody the frequency of LOVE at any given moment, even when we are in pain, surely we can give and receive love without fear of it "running out" or being "taken away."

Maybe the opening of your heart is as simple as remembering that you get to decide in EVERY moment how you will feel and respond.

A NOTE ON COMPASSION – WHO TAUGHT YOU HOW TO LOVE YOURSELF?

A few years ago I was having an existential crisis about coaching and life and all the things. My coach at the time asked me if I had ever felt this way before and I ended up way back in my childhood and told her I think I'd always had these lingering feelings. She asked me how had adults responded to these depressive phases when I was a kid and what had I actually needed. Well, I felt into it and realised that people had always been impatient with these emotions in my life. I suppose it was because they could see the depth of my pain and were worried but felt powerless to do anything and so they just encouraged me to stuff the feelings down, suck it up, stop crying, move the fuck on, and stop being so goddamn sensitive.

What I actually needed was just someone to see me. Someone to tell me that it would all be okay, that there was nothing wrong with me, and that I could take as long as I needed to feel how I felt and they would still be there loving me when I was ready to come back out of my shell – so I did that for myself. I was patient and compassionate and it COMPLETELY changed how I moved forward in my life. I am now so much more compassionate and patient with myself AND with others because I know that not a lot of people have actually been given the space to feel their feelings to the depth and full extent that they needed to when they were a kid and so … when you can hold yourself in this way and be compassionate, love yourself even when you feel completely fucked up and broken, like a weight in the world and useless, then you will be impenetrable.

And if you're ready for some next level heart healing … go through The spiral, ha ha!

WHAT THE FUCK IS THE SPIRAL?

Just a quickie on this in case you've not heard of it. The Spiral is a modality that borrows from kinesiology and works by combining the scale of consciousness, chakra system, and spiral dynamics over seven sessions. It works by clearing the 22 key emotions that keep people stuck in their shit. If you want to know more about this process, check out the resources section at the back of this book.

CHAPTER 8
THE BONUS META CHAPTER – EGO DEATHS AND IDENTITY UPGRADES

I wasn't planning on writing this chapter when I first mapped out the book, but as I began the process it became obvious to me that this needs to be said and so here I am sharing it with you.

I've spoken about the body/mind connection throughout this book and writing it has been no exception. As I have stepped into this new identity – the person who writes books, for example – and as I have written these stories of the girl I used to be, I became a woman. That might sound odd and a bit dramatic and it is, but so am I and I think you get that by now!

It was a few weeks before I began the physical writing process that the shifts began. I started to have these new awarenesses drop in around how I had still been feeling like I am just a kid (currently 36 as I write this) and maybe it is the Western way of having no real rites of passage (other than going out once a year and getting shit faced and I don't even do that anymore!). There is nothing that signifies to us that we have become WOMEN. Yes, we start to bleed around our teens and then we are legally allowed to have sex, etc. but these are such surface-level tokens that don't go anywhere near scratching the surface of what it really means to go from being a girl, a child who needs to ask others to help and even be rescued because she "doesn't know any better," to becoming the woman who has learned, grown, been burnt in the fires of her own mistakes and come back time and time again with a fresh perspective on the world.

There is no rite of passage for us and so maybe this book has been mine.

Two weeks before I started I got smacked down with the actual flu. The day I began writing I got a stye in my left eye – I have NEVER had one of these before and it is a pain in my ass ... well, it's a pain in my eye, actually, but y'get me.

As I am one to practise what I preach, my first instinct was to ask the stye what it was trying to tell me. This is what it said when I put pen to paper:

I'm sad. I'm sad for her and for you. I feel like you've forgotten the girl you left behind.
The one who wept her tears and felt the pain of losing him and in doing so felt the pain of losing her innocence.
He took it from me. Stripped me of my innocence. That's what men have done to me my whole life.
I have given myself willingly. I have offered myself up to the emotional slaughter time and time again and yet now I feel numb. Too afraid to feel the pain of my desires. Shutting myself down.
What else do you want me to know, little stye?
I'm here to hurt you. To feel discomfort. You need to be reminded of the pain so you can write about it.
And it is so sad. So much sadness in this little eye. This eye that has cried so many tears for so many boys who could not feel their own pain.

Intense, right?

The body wants to speak. It wants to be heard. The more we still ourselves and listen to what it is trying to communicate with us, the less we will suffer.

I have a daily energy clearing process that I use as well as journalling and movement when I feel called, but even just taking 10 minutes of your day to tune in and learn to listen to your beautiful body will change your life if you heed her words.

Anyway, back to the ego death/identity shift of writing this book.

After I had written the message from my stye I really felt that all the emotions I had been experiencing had been me resisting truly letting her go.

If I no longer have this story to refer back to or as a jumping-off point, what does that mean for me? Who will I become once my story is told and now I get to create this whole new life for myself beyond the confines of the past?

Writing this book has been an initiation and my hope is that reading it has been one for you too.

Living this life of constant soul expansion and transformation is not for the faint of heart or the despondent. We who choose this path must be bold, brave, and often ruthless in our pursuit of what lies ahead because we think it would be easy to just stop and stay where we are but we can't! The more we resist our own growth, the more it hurts.

The only way to ease the ego deaths you will encounter along the way is to SURRENDER (which is why I have it tattooed on my hand).

Being a recovering control freak, I have had a fractious relationship with surrender. I have learnt that only when you are truly ready to give up, let it go, carry on with life even if you don't get, do, or become the thing … only then are you truly ready to receive that for which you have been asking.

CHAPTER 9
SOUL SMACKDOWN – SO NOW WHAT?

Well, here we are, the final chapter! Anyone else say that to the tune of Europe's "Final Countdown"? No? Just me then.

If you made it this far you are clearly an epic badass and deserve a slice of cake and a spa day. You rule!

However, what happens now? Now that you've devoured this book and the nuggets within, what will you do?

Are you willing to do whatever it takes to shift out of overwhelm, powerlessness, and stagnation and stake a claim on the creation of your life?

Will this be another book on the bookshelf, possibly even one you rave about to friends (here's hopin'!), but how will you go about embodying the shifts that have occurred during your consumption of these concepts?

What we have awoken here is not just going to lay down and go back to sleep. You are AWAKE to what lives in your soul and you have everything you need to bring those dreams to life.

I know you SAY you want empowerment and freedom and to no longer give any fucks about what other people think, but are you truly ready to do what it takes to step into the spotlight and become the star of your own life?

If you can feel the fire in your belly building to a FUCK, YES … read on. Here are some helpful ways to break this shit down so you don't overwhelm yourself with your own badassery!

Own Your Desires: Get radically honest with yourself about what you want. What is working and what is not. Where in your life currently do you need to shake shit up and make some bold moves, speak some spicy truths, or just take the leap of faith and say yes to your soul?
One little nugget on why people, maybe even YOU, resist their desires. You have spent so long denying what you want by what hurts the least or what is the opposite of the thing that causes you pain and then you do this kind of transformational release and identity upgrade work and you no longer have those same reference points. Now you have to TRULY own what you want and without any of your former defence mechanisms, it's a bit fucking confusing.

When you KNOW that anything you want and everything you could possibly wish for is indeed available for you, it can be fucking terrifying! That is exactly what I am here for. I want to help you traverse these fears and the disorientation of change so that we can anchor you into creating the life you truly desire and deserve.

You may need to leave things and people behind. Are you ready to commit to this path even if it means you feel alone for a while? A big part of the growth journey is the bridge between the two worlds. Where you journey from where you are now – safe and sound and stuck in your rut, but it is comfy and cosy and familiar even if it does feel a bit restrictive and stagnant sometimes – to the in-between. The grey zone where it can feel as though you're wading through thick fog, totally alone without a torch to guide you, and you just have to TRUST that if you keep taking steps forward there is a whole host of next-level soul tribe on the other side waiting to welcome you with open arms?

I know how terrifying and lonely this sounds and honestly, there's no way to sugar-coat this … it is shit. However, it is SO worth it!! Now that you've cleaned up your vibration, taken full self-responsibility, and will be using that mirror like a goddamn BOSS, you will begin to attract friends like that too. I didn't even believe this was possible. I had done so much body clearing and mindset work around friendship over the years and nothing really stuck until I went through The Spiral in 2018 and then trained as a practitioner in the modality in February 2019 and met what I can only describe as my absolute soulmate friends.

When you waiver on your quest to fulfilment and freedom, you will falter because you are human and in those moments it will be really valuable to remember and reconnect to WHY you began in the first place. It is all too easy to look back over our shoulder with the rose-tinted glasses of nostalgia and think things used to be better. They weren't. Your ego is trying to squash you back into your safe little box where it can hold you hostage for another 30 years … No. Keep your eyes and heart focused on what you are calling in and who you are becoming and you will ease any transitions.

You have seen yourself in me, and now it is time to bring it home. If I can do it so can you! When I was writing this book, I asked my peeps what they wanted me to include in this book. They wanted to know what I am planning, moving forward!

So, what is next for me? Well, from here on I have a pretty good grounding for whatever I want to create in my life, but my real mission at this point is to get this message into the hands, ears, and hearts of as many people as possible! I want to reach millions of women just like YOU. Women who have a fire inside them about which they'd forgotten. I want to remind you and them of what you already know, but dare not trust. That YOU are a powerful force of nature and the world better watch out because you are coming for it!

ACKNOWLEDGEMENTS

- Francis Huelin – where do I begin? You have been my greatest teacher and I carry you in my heart always.

- Sara Wagstaffe – for introducing me to energy work and holding me so completely through my healing.

- John Daly – for supporting me on all my crazy whims and always believing in my magick.

- Heinz Longbody – you taught me how to love unconditionally.

- Jamy Schumacher and Kelly Grignon – for holding me accountable to my highest purpose and never letting me forget how goddamn powerful I am.

- And last but not least – Dave Thompson and Davina Davidson of Inspirational Book Writers. Without you I may never have got these words out of my body and into the world. Thank you for your unwavering support and belief in me. I LOVE YOU!

RESOURCES

Throughout this book I have mentioned several courses, modalities, books, and techniques.

To find out more about all of these resources, please go to: www.georginanoel.com/bookresources

ABOUT THE AUTHOR

Georgina Noel is passionate about helping women get out of their own way and being the permission to live a life of purpose and passion!

Through her work as a motivational speaker and mentor to creative, spiritual business owners, she assists driven badass women to activate shameless expression and soul expansion.

Georgina lives on the tiny island of Jersey in the Channel Islands where she spends the majority of her time training Muay Thai, drinking coffee, and stroking her mini Dachshund Heinz.

To find out more, go to: www.georginanoel.com
Email: hello@georginanoel.com
Facebook: @gnoelEFT
Instagram: @georginanoeleft

NOTES

NOTES

NOTES

NOTES

NOTES

NOTES

NOTES

NOTES

NOTES

NOTES

NOTES

Printed in Poland
by Amazon Fulfillment
Poland Sp. z o.o., Wrocław